The 15-Minute Standing Abs Workout Plan

Ten Simple Core Exercises to Firm, Tone, and Tighten Your Midsection

Second Edition
Dale L. Roberts
©2019

The 15-Minute Standing Abs Workout Plan: Ten Simple Core Exercises to Firm, Tone, and Tighten Your Midsection
All rights reserved
Original publication date October 17, 2015
Copyright ©2015 One Jacked Monkey, LLC
Second edition publication date May 15, 2019
All photos courtesy of Kelli Rae Roberts, October 2015

No part of this book may be reproduced or transmitted in any form or by any means, electronic or mechanical, including photocopying, recording or by any information storage and retrieval system, without the permission in writing from One Jacked Monkey, LLC.

Disclaimer
This book proposes a program of exercise recommendations. However, all readers must consult a qualified medical professional before starting this or any other health & fitness program. As with any exercise program, if at any time you experience any discomfort, pain or duress of any sort, stop immediately and consult your physician. This book is intended for an audience that is free of any health condition, physical limitation or injury. The creators, producers, participants, advertisers, and distributors of this program disclaim any liabilities or losses in connection with the exercises or advice herein. Any equipment or workout area that is used should be thoroughly inspected ahead of use as free of danger, flaw or compromise. The user assumes all responsibility when performing any movements contained in this book and waives the equipment manufacturer, makers, and distributors of the equipment of all liabilities.

Table of Contents

Introduction 1
Benefits of These 10 Exercises 2
Standing Versus Sitting or Lying Down 3
Using More than Your Abs 4
What is the Core? 5
The 10 Standing Abs Exercises 7
    Stomach Flattener 8
    Knee-Ups 10
    Front & Back Bends 12
    Side Bends 14
    Waist Turners 16
    Standing Cross Crunch 18
    Helicopters 20
    Hands Together Side Bends 22
    Bend, Twist & Touch 24
    Trunk Rotations 26
The 15-Minute Standing Abs Workout Plan 28
The Best Time to Use the Program 29
Conclusion 30
Thank You 31
About The Author 32
Special Thanks 33
References 34

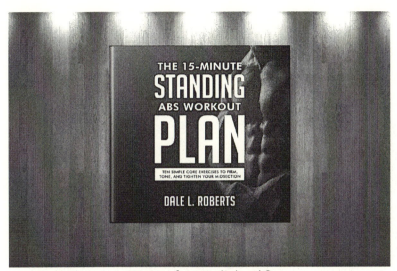

Want a free audiobook?
Would you like to have a full abs workout plan?
Then, get a free copy of *The 15-Minute Standing Abs Workout Plan*...
When you get a free 30-day trial of Audible at this link:
US - DaleLRoberts.com/Abs
UK - DaleLRoberts.com/AbsUK
Germany - DaleLRoberts.com/AbsDE
France - DaleLRoberts.com/AbsFR

Introduction

When I was a personal trainer, I received a lot of requests to tone up and firm the mid-section. So, *The 15-Minute Standing Abs Workout Plan* is my best solution to easily accommodate most everyone. This book is for anyone looking to use effective abs exercises, regardless of their fitness experience. Whether you're a beginner or an athlete, if you can stand, then you should be able to perform these exercises.

Rather than spend tons of money and time on fancy exercise equipment, you have these exercises wherever you go and use them whenever you want. These standing abs exercises are excellent as active recovery between sets during a workout or as a standalone workout.

In fact, these exercises are my morning routine and combine for a tremendous go-to workout when I'm pressed for time. Doing these exercises gets my blood pumping, my energy revitalized and my day kick-started in a significant way. If you're new to working out in the morning, give these exercises a shot.

I won't make outrageous claims or promise you stellar results from these exercises. However, if you incorporate these recommendations into a daily routine, you'll feel good about yourself, carry yourself better and feel accomplished once you master them.

Benefits of These 10 Exercises

When performed daily, the 10 standing abs exercises bring some advantages including:

1. A firmer midsection
2. Definition and muscle tone in the core area
3. More lung power
4. More stamina in athletic activities
5. Less risk of injury

Standing Versus Sitting or Lying Down

You burn more calories when you're standing than when sitting or lying down. When you stand, you have to activate more muscles than when you're seated or lying. If you want to get the most from your exercises, then do them standing instead of sitting or lying.

In a recent summary of a 12-year study held at the Pennington Biomedical Research Center, the association between daily standing time and death among 16,586 adults revealed standing may not be dangerous to your health. In fact, the risk of death significantly decreased with higher levels of standing as opposed to excessive sitting.[i] This seems rather simple information everyone should know, right? Exactly!

This report further confirms what we've suspected all along. Standing is far better for your health as opposed to sitting. With the 10 standing abs exercises, you'll implement movements from a standing position to strengthen your mobility or your ability to move or walk. It only makes sense if you want to function better while standing, then you should work out from a standing position. In my opinion, it's highly unlikely that writhing about on the floor will do much good for your ability to stand and function from a standing position. So, stick with what sets you up for the greatest success. Stand up and exercise.

Hey, let's face it. It's not always fun to get down to the floor when you have to do a few sets of an abs exercise. Afterward, you still have to get back up to your feet. Though most active adults may not find getting up and down an inconvenience, there are some who find this movement difficult. Eliminate the extraneous work and simply stay on your feet. Then, when you have built more strength and stamina, floor exercises are complimentary to your normal exercise routine.

Using More than Your Abs

Isolated training, or specifically targeting one muscle group for exercise, isn't all it's cracked up to be. Unless you're a fitness or bodybuilding competitor, targeting one muscle in a workout isn't functional in your everyday life. You need something better suited to your lifestyle. And, the exercises need to serve multiple functions when you do them, such as:

1. Burn calories – all exercises burn calories which, in turn, burns fat so you get the lean figure you've always wanted.
2. Saves time – exercising should fit your schedule, so you should do something with a reasonable time investment.
3. Have the most benefits – any exercise you perform should get the most results in the least time. When you utilize more muscle, you burn more calories.
4. Be safe – any workout you do shouldn't compromise your safety.
5. Be functional – exercise should mimic movement you would normally do throughout your day to move more efficiently and possibly decrease the risk of injury.

Though this book's title insinuates only ab exercises, the 10 movements do more than isolate your abdominal muscles. When done correctly, each exercise trains a part of the core. The exercises in this book build a solid midsection while strengthening your spine in the process. And, these results have far more long-term benefits than just abs-specific training.

What is the Core?

These days, when it comes to health and fitness, the word "core" is thrown around a lot. However, few people seem to know what the core is and how it pertains to their health. Additionally, once someone has a basic understanding of what the core is, not too many people know how to train it effectively.

The core, also known as the trunk, is all the major muscles that move, support and stabilize your spine. This area includes the abdominal muscles from the front of your body wrapping all the way around to the back. This includes the smaller muscles along the spinal column that aid in stabilizing and keeping your body upright.

The core muscles help you bend forward, stand upright, bend backward and sideways, twist, draw your stomach in and stabilize your spine during any movement. The overall development of your core determines what you can accomplish in your workouts. The 10 standing abs exercises address the core in many functions and directions, getting the most advantages for your core from a standing position.

The 10 Standing Abs Exercises

I share links for each exercise to videos on YouTube where you can follow along. Sadly, you don't have the convenience of simply clicking the link in this print book like you would in an ebook. However, I took the liberty of cleaning up the long URL and kept it memorable and simple. Bookmark the video in your browser so you can return to it later. If you have any questions or need any modifications, feel free to drop a comment on the video and I'll answer you as soon as possible.

Stomach Flattener

Follow along with the video at this link: DaleLRoberts.com/Abs1

1. Place your fingers spread out on your stomach below your ribs. Use your fingertips to ensure you're tightening your abs during this exercise.
2. Take a deep breath in through your nose and allow your stomach to expand. Then, tighten your stomach as tight as possible at the peak of your breath.
3. Briefly pause, and then slowly and forcefully exhale through your mouth.
4. Continue to tighten your stomach and do not stop breathing out until you've fully exhaled. You should have to inhale immediately afterward if you do this exercise correctly.

NOTE: It's not unusual to feel slightly light-headed after this exercise. However, do not continue the stomach flattener if the symptom persists.

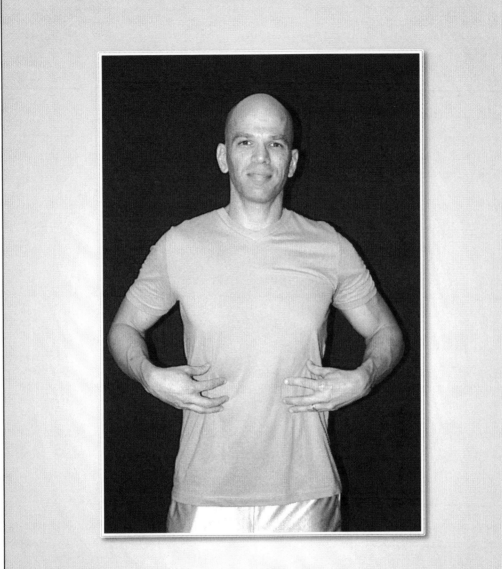

Knee-Ups

Follow along with the video at this link: DaleLRoberts.com/Abs2

1. Stagger your stance, placing your weight on the lead foot.
2. Raise your back heel. Put your hands overhead.
3. Bring your hands down while driving your rear knee up to meet in the middle.
4. Quickly return to the starting position.

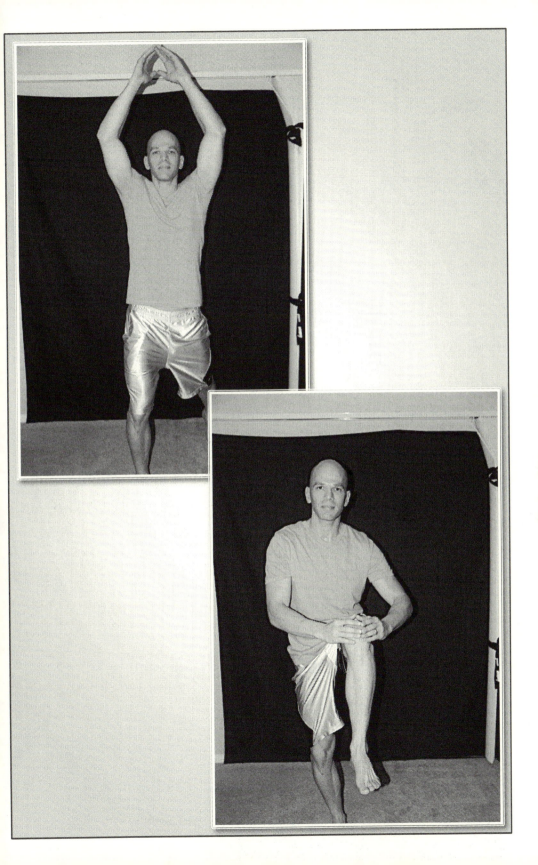

Front & Back Bends

Follow along with the video at this link: DaleLRoberts.com/Abs3

1. Place your hands on your hips. Bend at the waist as far forward as you can go.
2. Pause in this position and squeeze your abs for a 3-count.
3. Come back up to a full standing position.
4. Bend back as far as you can go, then immediately return to the start position.

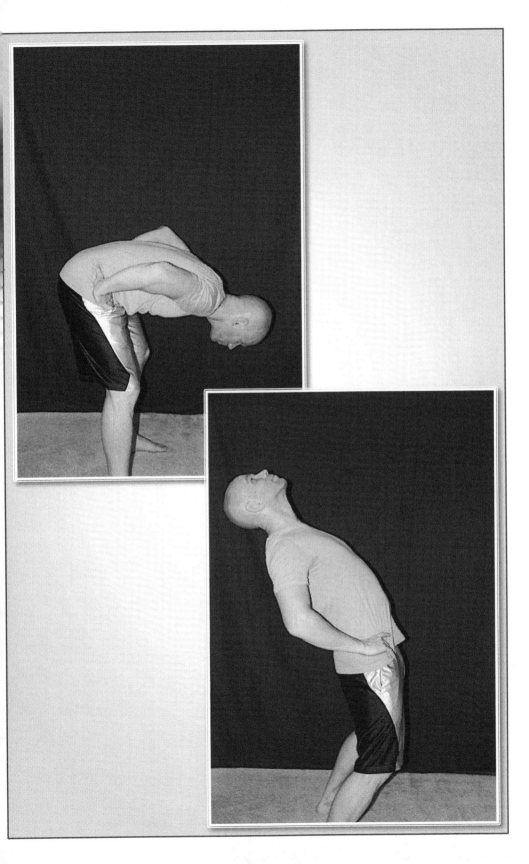

Side Bends

Follow along with the video at this link: DaleLRoberts.com/Abs4

1. Extend one arm overhead and keep the other arm by your side.
2. Bend your body directly to the side.
3. Allow the downward arm to slide along your thigh until you can't go any further.
4. Bring your body upright while tightening your mid-section.

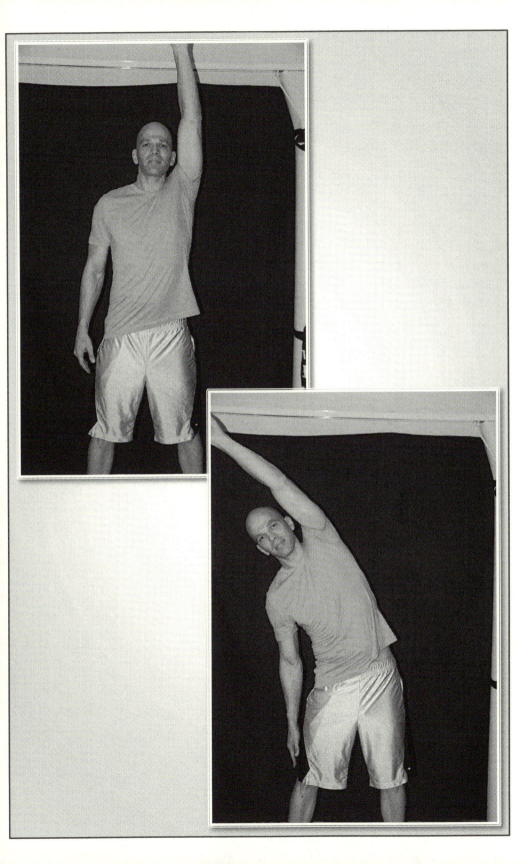

Waist Turners

Follow along with the video at this link: DaleLRoberts.com/Abs5

1. Allow your arms to loosely hang at your sides and separate your feet shoulder-width apart.
2. Keep your feet flat on the floor throughout the exercise.
3. Turn your upper body to the left, then to the right.
4. Repeat this sequence, allowing your arms to turn with the movement. As momentum increases, your hands will simultaneously slap at the mid- to lower-back area.
5. Keep a controlled movement throughout and avoid snapping quickly from one side to the other.

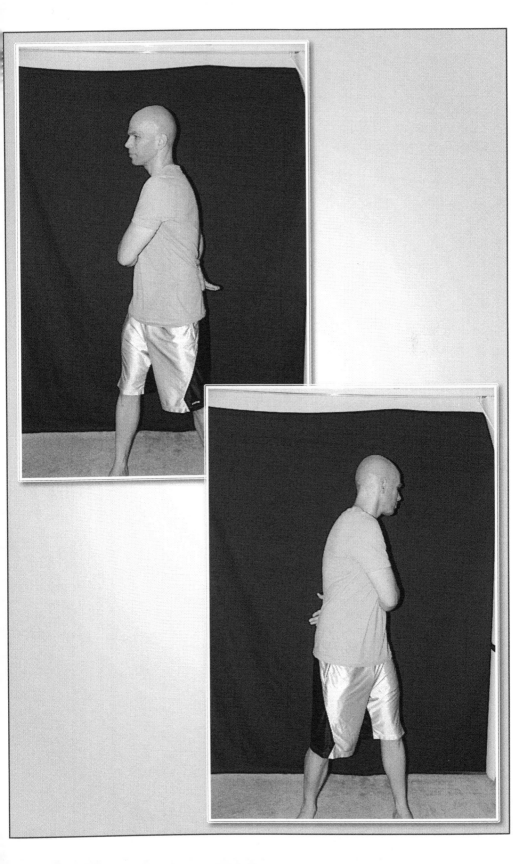

Standing Cross Crunch

Follow along with the video at this link: DaleLRoberts.com/Abs6

1. Separate your feet shoulder-width apart and stagger your stance.
2. Place your hands behind your head and pull your elbows back.
3. Draw your rear knee up and the opposite elbow down to meet together.
4. Squeeze your abs in this position.
5. Then, return to the starting position.
6. Now repeat the movement on the opposite side.

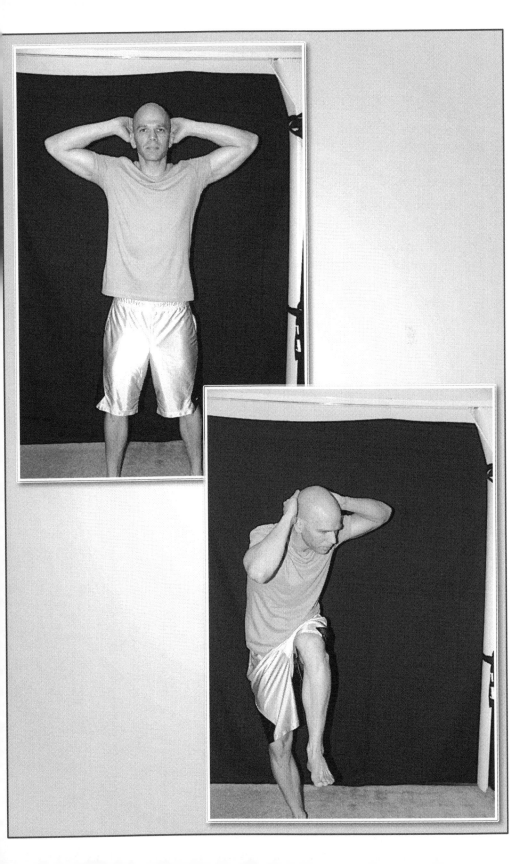

Helicopters

Follow along with the video at this link: DaleLRoberts.com/Abs7

1. Separate your feet shoulder-width apart and extend your arms at your shoulders.
2. Rotate at your torso, pop up your heel and pivot on the ball of the foot you turn away from.
3. When you have reached the farthest point, tighten your abs.
4. Return to the starting position.
5. Repeat the movement sequence in the other direction.

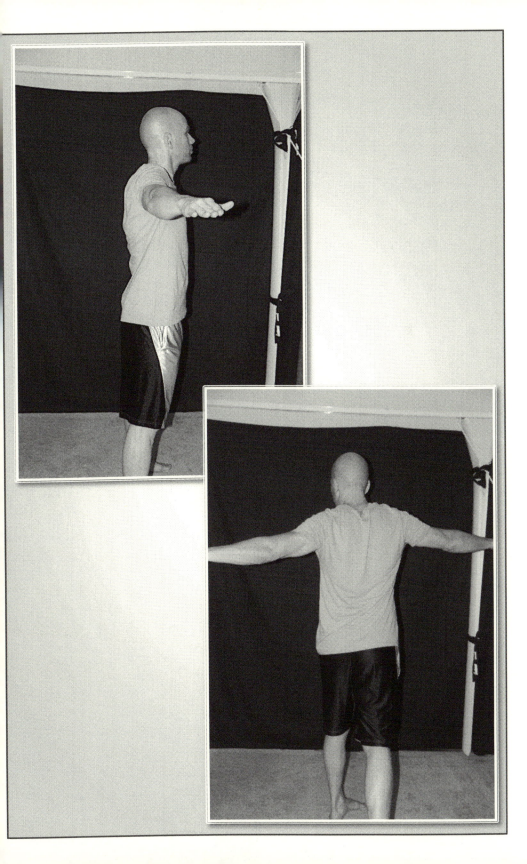

Hands Together Side Bends

Follow along with the video at this link: DaleLRoberts.com/Abs8

1. Interlace your fingers and extend your arms overhead with your palms up.
2. Bend to one side as far as you can go and hold for a 5-count.
3. Tighten your mid-section and bring yourself upright.
4. Repeat the movement sequence on the other side.

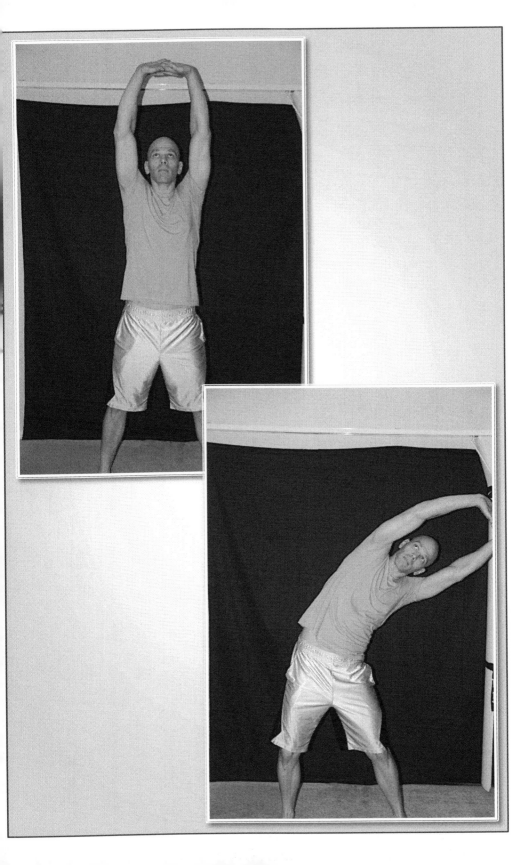

Bend, Twist & Touch

Follow along with the video at this link: DaleLRoberts.com/Abs9

1. Separate your feet wider than shoulder-width apart.
2. Extend your arms out from your shoulders.
3. Bend at your waist and turn your torso to the left.
4. Touch your left foot with your right hand; squeeze your abs for a 1- to 3-count.
5. Return to the starting position.
6. Repeat the movement sequence on the opposite side.

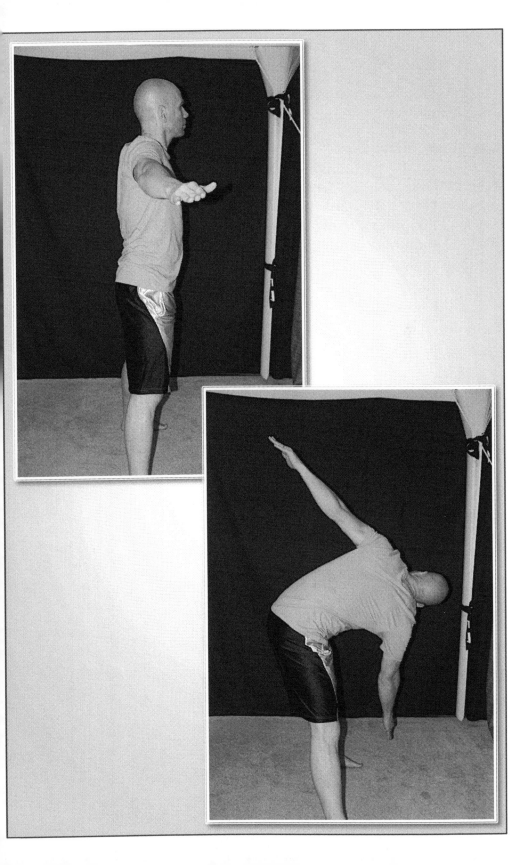

Trunk Rotations

Follow along with the video at this link: DaleLRoberts.com/Abs10

1. Place your hands on your hips.
2. Bend at the waist as far forward as you can go.
3. Then, slowly rotate from one side to the other.
4. Think of drawing a large circle with your upper body as you rotate around.

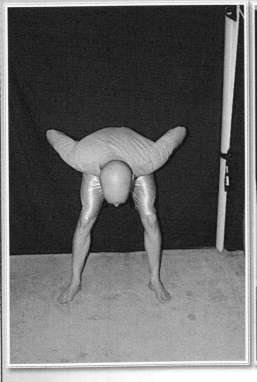
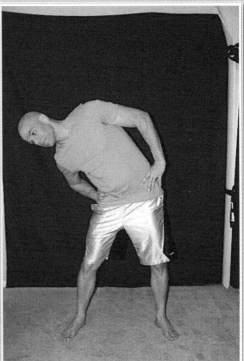
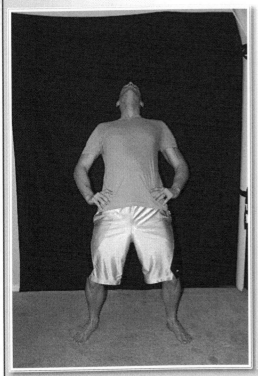
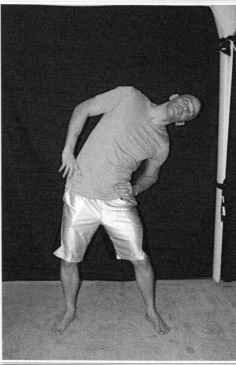

The 15-Minute Standing Abs Workout Plan

Now, string together these exercises for a short and practical 15-minute workout. Follow along with the video at this link: DaleLRoberts.com/TotalAbs

1 - Stomach Flattener for 1 minute
2 - Knee-ups for 1 minute
3 - Front & Back Bends for 2 minutes
4 - Side Bends for 1 minute each side (2 minutes total)
5 - Waist Turners for 1 minute
6 – Standing Cross Crunch for 1 minute each side (2 minutes total)
7 - Helicopters for 1 minute
8 - Hands Together Side Bends for 2 minutes
9 - Bend, Twist & Touch for 1 minute
10 - Trunk Rotations for 1 minute each direction (2 minutes total)

The Best Time to Use the Program

The ideal time for this exercise routine is right after you wake up. Make sure you're fully awake before you jump into this routine. Begin the routine slow while gradually picking up your pace and extending the range you do them.

If you are pressed for time, then do what you can before getting into your day. When I have missed my morning abs routine, I try to make it up by using the exercises between sets in a workout. You can catch your breath between intense exercise sets and keep your core activated with the 10 exercises in this book.

Here are some general guidelines for you to choose according to your fitness level:
• Beginner or Returning to Exercise – 1-3 times per week
• Experienced – 4-7 times per week – as much as daily
• Athletes – 2 times per day – right when you wake up and as a warm-up to any exercise routine

Conclusion

Time is the most valuable and precious resource in life. And, you don't always have the luxury to relax and get your workout in, too. When pressed for time, you should always opt for getting in something. Any activity is better than nothing at all. I don't need to point to peer-reviewed scientific studies for you to agree on one thing. Staying active keeps you healthier than being sedentary or doing little to nothing at all.

I'm confident the 10 standing abs exercises will serve you well if you take just 15 minutes out of your day to do them. Once you finish, you will be glad you did. And then you can carry on with whatever else life throws at you.

Use *The 15-Minute Standing Abs Workout Plan* for the next month, and I'll bet you'll see and feel the difference. Take a starting measurement around your midsection on your first day. Then, re-measure every 30 days to track your progress.

Remember, this program isn't a quick fix. You'll see gradual results if using the workout plan consistently. As always, if you need to lose excess weight, be sure to eat mindfully. Avoid processed foods and fast food restaurants as much as you can. Eat plenty of whole foods such as green leafy vegetables and fruits. And, if you afford the time, consider a weight training program to expedite your results. The World Health Organization suggests adults exercise at least 75 to 150 minutes throughout the week. [ii] Consult your family doctor for appropriate activities according to your health needs.

Whatever you choose to do, I hope you make a choice to become healthier by the day, challenge yourself and become a stronger human being. It really is simple to get into great shape since it takes only one step at a time. I'm confident this book delivers an easy, cost-effective solution for anyone. All you have to do is put it into practice. Now, stand up. And, for the next 15 minutes, start exercising!

Thank You

Thank you for reading this book, and I hope you enjoyed it. As you work toward your health and fitness goals, you may have questions or run into some issues. I'd like to be able to help you, so let's connect. Feel free to reach out to me online at:
• Website: DaleLRoberts.com
• YouTube: YouTube.com/PTDaleLRoberts
• Facebook: Facebook.com/AuthorDaleRoberts
• Follow me on Twitter: Twitter.com/PTDaleRoberts

Thank you, again! I hope to hear from you and wish you the best.

Want a free audiobook?
Would you like to have a **full** workout plan?
Then, get a free copy of *The 90-Day Home Workout Plan*...
When you get a free 30-day trial of Audible at this link:
US - DaleLRoberts.com/90dayUS
UK - DaleLRoberts.com/90dayUK
France - DaleLRoberts.com/90dayFrance
Germany - DaleLRoberts.com/90dayGermany

About The Author

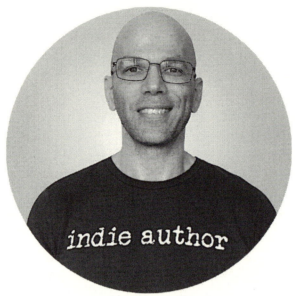

Dale L. Roberts is an experienced indie author, self-publishing expert and former personal trainer. While Dale loves to share his passion and enthusiasm for health and fitness, his greatest love is helping other people realize their dreams and live life on their terms. He currently lives with his wife, Kelli, in Columbus, Ohio.

Special Thanks

None of my fitness books would be possible without the undying support of my beautiful wife, Kelli. She's been my biggest cheerleader, greatest coach and best friend in the whole process.

I also owe a debt of gratitude to my subscriber base on the *Self-Publishing with Dale* YouTube Channel. You help me keep it real, stay grounded and strive to be better. Not to mention, my core peeps including Kevin Maguire, Keith Wheeler, Mojo Siedlak, Mark Brownless, Risa Fey and all the folks in the Self-Publishing Books Group on Facebook. You guys are my fam!

And, lastly, YOU, the reader. Even after selling thousands of books over the past five years, I still feel like I owe you better content with every new release or update. Hence why I decided to pull the first edition of this book and refine the content. I hope you enjoyed this book as much as I did when updating it.

References

[i] Katzmarzyk PT. (2014). Standing and mortality in a prospective cohort of Canadian adults. Retrieved on 2015, October 16 from http://www.ncbi.nlm.nih.gov/pubmed/24152707

[ii] World Health Organization. (n.d.). Physical Activity and Adults. Retrieved on 2015, October 17 from http://www.who.int/dietphysicalactivity/factsheet_adults/en/

Made in the USA
Middletown, DE
08 September 2020